HEPATIC HORIZON

A CLINICAL GUIDE TO LIVER
DISEASE MANAGEMENT

DR. EDWARD NICHOLAS

Copyright

Copying or reproducing this book without the author's permission is prohibited (© 2024).

TABLE OF CONTENT

INTRODUCTION 5
CHAPTER 1 9
   NON-ALCOHOLIC LIVER DISEASE (NAFLD) 9
CHAPTER 2 22
CIRRHOSIS 22
CHAPTER 3 46
   HEMOCHROMATOSIS 46
CHAPTER 4 61
   HEPATITIS B 61
CHAPTER 5 76
   HEPATITIS C 76
1. Acute Hepatitis C: 80
2. Chronic Hepatitis C: 81
1. Antiviral Therapy: 83
2. Monitoring and Supportive Care: 84
3. Liver Transplantation: 84
CHAPTER 6 89
   PRIMARY BILIARY CHOLANGITIS (PBC) 89
1. Prevalence: 90
2. Incidence: 90
3. Gender Distribution: 90
4. Age of Onset: 91
5. Geographical Variation: 91
6. Risk Factors: 91
7. Ethnic Differences: 92
CHAPTER 7 105
   PRIMARY SCLEROSING CHOLANGITIS (PSC) 105
1. Medical Therapy: 114
2. Endoscopic and Surgical Interventions: 115
3. Management of Associated Conditions: 116
7 DAY DIETARY PLAN FOR PSC 116
CONCLUSION 120

INTRODUCTION

Liver disease can be best described as the medical condition that involves the liver which can be defined as an vital internal organ in the human body that is responsible for number of functions including detoxification, synthesis of proteins and generation of essential biochemicals for digestion. The liver regenerates itself but the organ is prone to numerous ailments that reduce its ability to perform its work and cause life-threatening effects.

The diseases of the liver can be classified according to the cause: viral hepatitis; inherited liver disease; auto-immune disease; and diseases that are probably linked with a person's lifestyle issue such as alcohol drinking, obesity and more. The common liver diseases include cirrhosis, liver cancer, viral hepatitis, chronic hepatitis B and C, steatohepatitis, NAFLD, and alcoholic liver disease. The book highlights that NAFLD is increasingly prevalent, particularly in developed countries, and may be entwined with metabolic syndrome, diabetes, obesity. This means that it is not about the accumulation of alcohol within liver cells, and it can cause more severe liver health conditions such as cirrhosis, liver cancer, and Non-alcoholic steatohepatitis (NASH).Alcoholism leads to the development of Alcoholic Liver Disease (ALD), which can range from simple steatosis to exacerbated alcoholic hepatitis, fibrosis, and cirrhosis. With regular use of alcohol for a long term time, alcohol damages the liver and is thus a primary cause of the condition. Viral hepatitis is also a prevalent type of liver disease in the world today; it is caused by Hepatitis B and C viruses. If they are left untreated these infections reach the state of chronic diseases that lead to development of serious complications such as cirrhosis and liver cancer. The controversies related to the employment of vaccinations and antiviral medications have been vital in containing the consequences and transmission of these infections. Chronic liver illnesses such as hepatitis and ALD can lead to cirrhosis, which is characterized by permanent scarring of the liver. It damages the liver, increases the chance of liver cancer, and can cause liver failure.

Liver disease is also influenced by genetic conditions including Wilson's disease and hemochromatosis. If left untreated, hemochromatosis and Wilson's disease both result in excessive iron and copper buildup in the liver, respectively, which can cause damage to the liver.

The immune system attacks the liver or bile ducts in autoimmune disorders such as Primary Sclerosing Cholangitis (PSC) and

Primary Biliary Cholangitis (PBC), resulting in persistent inflammation and scarring. Liver disease is ubiquitous as evidenced by the fact that millions of people are affected by the diseases and the conditions result in a lot of morbidity and mortality. The key to stopping the development of liver diseases or to fa our a patient ' s prognosis lies in the accurate identification of the disease at an early stage. Hence, the role of public health promotion and early interventions including immunization, health promotion and awareness on lifestyles, and early detection programs are paramount in the prevention and management of liver diseases.

CHAPTER 1

NON-ALCOHOLIC LIVER DISEASE (NAFLD)

NAFLD or Non-Alcoholic Fatty Liver Disease is one of the conditions that involve the buildup of fat in the liver of a person who hardly drinks alcohol or does not drink at all. This illness is now an emerging problem in many parts of the world especially in the developed nations owing to its linkages to obesity, diabetes, and metabolic syndrome . NAFLD includes simple steatosis, steatohepatitis and NASH progressing to cirrhosis, liver failure, and liver cancer.

EPIDEMIOLOGY

1. Approximately one quarter to one third of the global population is affected by NAFLD, which is considered to be the most common liver condition in the world at the present time. The

prevalence of this condition is markedly higher in metabolic syndrome, type 2 diabetics, and the obese population. A preliminary survey indicates that between 30 and 40% of adults in the United States has NAFLD; higher prevalence has been observed in certain races or ethnicities such as Hispanic population. The same seems to apply to Australia and the United Kingdom, where increased obesity and diabetes tendencies increase the scope of NAFLD as well.

PATHOPHYSIOLOGY

The etiology of NAFLD is multifactorial and complex as many factors can lead to the development of this disease. Among the crucial elements in its pathophysiology are:

1. **Insulin resistance:** Insulin resistance is a central feature of NAFLD. Enhanced lipolysis is the result and

this in turn raises the concentration of FFA's in the blood since they are liberated from the adipose tissue. Because of this fatty acids are absorbed by the liver leading to fat accumulation.

2. **Oxidative stress:** The excessive fat in the liver results in increased production of ROS which leads to oxidation stress and inflammation. This can affect liver cells leading to development of NASH from simple steatosis.

3. **Inflammation:** The development of nonalcoholic fatty liver disease (NAFLD) is significantly influenced by the production of adipokines and inflammatory cytokines from LDL and adipose tissue. Hepatic cell damage, fibrosis, and cirrhosis can result from chronic inflammation.

4. **Gut microbiota:** NAFLD has been linked to changes in the gut microbiota. A dysbiosis (an

unbalanced population of gut bacteria) can cause an increase in gut permeability, which can then cause bacterial endotoxins to go into the liver and cause inflammation.

RISK FACTORS

The onset of NAFLD is influenced by multiple risk factors which include:

Obesity: Excess body weight, Especially central obesity is a major risk factor for NAFLD.

Type 2 Diabetes: Individuals with type 2 diabetes are at increased risk of NAFLD.

Metabolic Syndrome: a set of conditions hypertension, hyperlipidemia, and insulin resistance.

Genetics: Genetic predisposition: Some gene variants are actually related to an increased risk of NAFLD

Inactivity/sedentary lifestyle: Being inactive can be a risk factor.

Diet: Diet is associated with NAFLD as diets are high in fructose, fats and sugar; in particular there seems to be an association with diets high in fructose, sugared beverages, and saturated fats.

CLINICAL FEATURES

Early NAFLD is frequently asymptomatic and hard to recognize. If symptoms occur, they may include:

Fatigue: One of the most common symptoms in people with NAFLD.

Right Upper Abdominal Pain: Some patients suffer from mild right upper abdominal pain or discomfort.

Hepatomegaly: On physical examination, moderate hepatomegaly may be noted.

In addition to these mild symptoms, there are some others that could occur as the disease advances to NASH and cirrhosis. Some examples of such symptoms include: *Jaundice* (yellowing of the skin and eyes). *Ascites* (accumulation of fluid in the abdomen). *Edema* (swelling in the legs and ankles). *Hepatic Encephalopathy* (in this condition, people become confused due to liver failure as well as cognitive impairment).

DIAGNOSIS

Clinical assessment, blood testing, imaging scans, and occasionally a liver biopsy are used to diagnose non-alcoholic fatty liver disease (NAFLD):

1. **Clinical Evaluation:** Evaluation for risk factors such as obesity, diabetes, and metabolic syndrome.

2. **Laboratory Tests:** Blood work to assess liver enzymes (ALT, AST), lipid profile, fasting glucose, and HbA1c.

3. **Imaging Studies:** The most common test used to detect liver fat is ultrasound. Other imaging techniques, including MRI and FibroScan, can provide additional information on liver fat and fibrosis.

4. **Liver Biopsy:** This is the gold standard for diagnosing NASH and for evaluation of fibrosis; however, this is an invasive procedure, and biopsies are not performed routinely.

MANAGEMENT

1. **Pharmacotherapy:**
   - **Insulin Sensitizers**: Metformin and thiazolidinediones (including pioglitazone) can be prescribed to enhance the action of insulin.

   - **Lipid-Lowering Agents**: Lipid-lowering agents such as statins should be considered in patients with dyslipidemia.

   - **Vitamin E:** In some situations, antioxidant therapy with vitamin E may be useful especially if the patient does not have diabetes mellitus and has NASH.

2. **Bariatric Surgery:** Bariatric surgery may be an option for those with severe obesity and NAFLD who do not respond to lifestyle changes. It has been demonstrated to improve liver histology and cause a notable reduction in body weight.

3.**Management of commodities:** In order to treat NAFLD holistically, control of diabetes, hypertension, and hyperlipidemia is crucial.

4.**Lifestyle changes:**
- **Weight Loss**: Life-style modification, specifically changes in diet and increased exercise are an important part of NAFLD treatment with weight loss preferred to be slow and steady. Based on a number of types ofdiet it is possible to achieve only an insignificant decrease in body weight, but it will be enough to achieve a reduction in hepatic steatosis and inflammation by 5- 10%.

- **Physical Activity**: Consistent exercise, including resistance and aerobic training, helps lower liver fat and enhance insulin sensitivity.

- **Diet**: Refined Carbs, fructose and saturated fats should then be consumed in limited quantities and this should be accompanied by a healthy diet. As part of an empirical nocturnal dietary intervention, the Mediterranean diet has emerged as beneficial in the case of NAFLD due to its emphasis on fruits and vegetables, whole grains, and healthy fats.

7-DAY DIET PLAN FOR NON - ALCOHOLIC FATTY LIVER DISEASE

DAYS	BREAKFAST	LUNCH	DINNER
DAY 1	Smoothie with spinach, banana, almond milk, protein powder, and flaxseeds	Quinoa bowl with black beans, corn, bell peppers, and lime	Stir-fried tofu with mixed vegetables and brown rice
DAY 2	Oatmeal with berries and	Grilled chicken	Baked salmon with

		chia seeds	salad with mixed greens and vinaigrette	steamed broccoli and sweet potato mash
DAY 3		Greek yogurt with granola and strawberries	Lentil soup with a side of whole-grain bread	Grilled turkey burger with a whole-grain bun, lettuce, tomato, and a side of sweet potato fries
DAY 4		Whole-grain toast with avocado and poached egg, mixed fruit	Turkey and avocado wrap with mixed greens	Lean beef stir-fry with bell peppers, snap peas, and quinoa
DAY 5		Oatmeal with sliced banana and a sprinkle of nuts	Mixed greens salad with grilled shrimp, tomatoes, cucumbers, and olive oil dressing	Baked chicken breast with quinoa and roasted vegetables
DAY 6		Smoothie bowl with	Chicken and vegetable	Baked cod with

	mixed berries, banana, and a sprinkle of granola	stir-fry with brown rice	steamed asparagus and quinoa
DAY 7	Whole-grain pancakes with a drizzle of honey and fresh fruit	Spinach and feta stuffed chicken breast with a side salad	Celery sticks with almond

PROGNOSIS

NAFLD has a guarded prognosis, which depends on the severity of the disease at the time of diagnosis and the persistence of other co-morbidities. Most cases of simple steatosis are benign but 20-30 % of these patients progress to NASH and these are at a higher risk of fibrosis cirrhosis, liver related complications, including Hepatocellular carcinoma. Screening and timely treatment are significant when is has to do with the progress of the actual disease or condition.

CONCLUSION

Non-Alcoholic Fatty Liver Disease is a prominent and emerging issue in modern society due to obesity and metabolic syndrome explosion all over the world. It is primarily asymptomatic in its early stages which hinders diagnosis and treatment. Knowledge in NAFLD risk factors, underlying mechanisms, and clinical manifestations are crucial in order to prevent, diagnose and manage NAFLD. These measures include change in diet, weight loss, and exercise remain the cornerstone of managing the conditions. More studies should be conducted to identify effective treatments and enhance the quality of life of patients living with such a common liver disorder. Community health strategies that are targeting awareness on improved lifestyles and early checks are important in the fight against a continuously increasing NAFLD burden.

CHAPTER 2

CIRRHOSIS

Liver cirrhosis is a long-term, continually deteriorating condition that involves the rebuilding of a significant part of the liver with scar tissue. This process is called fibrosis and can often hinder proper functioning of the liver and cause various serious consequences.

Liver cirrhosis is one of the most common liver diseases where the liver functions are impaired due to scarring brought about by the chronic destruction of liver cells. The liver, which forms the largest internal organ within the body, plays key roles in the body, including detoxification, bile production and storage of vitamins and minerals. Some of the functions of the liver involve repairing itself, but when this happens, scar tissues are produced when the liver is damaged. As the scarring increases over time, the liver's function diminishes due to obstruction of regular working. It is crucial to have an understanding of liver cirrhosis as it is a prevalent condition and an end-stage consequence of many chronic liver diseases affecting millions of people globally. It is hoped that this guide will offer a well-informed and easy to understand general understanding of liver cirrhosis, its development, its signs, its detection, its management, and how it can be treated or avoided.

EPIDEMIOLOGY
GLOBAL PREVALENCE
Millions of people throughout the world suffer from liver cirrhosis, a common health problem. Globally, liver cirrhosis ranks among the top 20 causes of death, according to the World Health Organization (WHO). About 1.3 million fatalities annually, or 2.4% of all deaths, are attributed to it. This substantial figure emphasizes how

important it is to raise awareness and take preventative action.

REGIONAL VARIATION

Liver cirrhosis is not uniform across the world because it is occasioned by different risks in different parts of the world.

1. **Asia**: Epidemiology of hepatitis B and C infections also shows that in many Asian countries cirrhosis of the liver is frequent complication. For instance, hepatitis B is quite rampant in China and this has considerably boosted the prevalence of liver diseases.

2. **Western Countries**: In the North American and European region, alcohol consumption and NAFLD are prominent causes. NAFLD is prevalent in the United States with approximately 30–40% of the adult population being affliction, and approximately 4. It is estimated that, 5

million people suffer from liver cirrhosis.

3. **Africa**: Hepatitis B especially is very prevalent in the sub-Saharan Africa, and has become the leading cause of liver cirrhosis in this area.

GENDER AND AGE

Liver cirrhosis is common in both sexes but with more presenting rates in the male gender. Many believe that such a gender divide results from higher alcohol intake among male drinkers. Moreover, liver cirrhosis is seen in people who are in the age group of fifty and above and can affect other age groups as well. It is for that reason that younger populations have not been left behind when it comes to NAFLD.

PATHOPHYSIOLOGY

The intricate process of liver cirrhosis culminates in the breakdown of liver function and increasing scarring, or fibrosis. It is brought on by a persistent injury to the liver from a variety of sources, including viral hepatitis, alcoholism, and non-alcoholic fatty liver disease (NAFLD). Examining how liver cells, or hepatocytes, and the structure of the liver are gradually harmed and changed is necessary to comprehend the pathophysiology of liver cirrhosis.

1.**Chronic Liver Injury:** Liver cirrhosis develops as follows, individuals experience persistent liver cell damage which causes inflammation. Common causes of chronic liver injury:
- Alcohol consumption
- Hepatitic viral diseases (Hepatitis B & C)
- Non alcoholic fatty liver disease or Non alcoholic steatohepatitis (NASH)
- Autoimmune hepatitis

- Iron overload diseases and other inherited diseases (examples: haemochromatosis, Wilson's disease

2. Inflammatory Response: In response to chronic injury, the liver undergoes inflammatory response:
- Kupffer cells (the macrophages of the liver) get activated and secrete pro-inflammatory cytokines.
- Damage to hepatocytes also causes the release of endogenous ligands that provoke inflammation as DAMPs.

3. Activation of Stellate Cells:
- In normal liver, stellate cells contain vitamin A and are inactive.
- These cells become activated in response to chronic injury and change their morphology into myofibroblast-like cells.
- Activated stellate cells make increased amounts of extracellular

matrix (ECM) molecules including collagen and therefore cause fibrosis.

4. **Fibrosis Formation:** The excessive ECM deposition by activated stellate cells leads to fibrosis:
- Liver fibrosis is characterized by the accumulation of excessive amount of collagens and other ECM molecules.
- It destroys the normal architecture of the liver and replaces healthy organic tissue by fibrous tissue which form fibrous septa that subdivide the liver into nodules.

5. **Vascular Changes:** The structural changes in cirrhotic liver lead to significant vascular alterations:
- Sinusoidal capillarization: The fenestrations constituent of the liver sinusoids are then eliminated, or remains narrow meaning that there is little inter-change between blood and hepatocytes.

- Intrahepatic resistance: Liver fibrosis associated with development of regenerative nodules raises the livers resistance to blood flow for the creation of portal hypertension.

6.**Portal Hypertension:** is a major complication of cirrhosis, characterized by increased pressure in the portal venous system:
- Increased intrahepatic resistance: As a result of liver fibrosis and regenerative nodules.
- Hyperdynamic circulation: Increased blood flow to the splanchnic (abdominal) organs to overcome mostly the resistance of the liver.

7. **Liver Dysfunction:** As cirrhosis progresses, liver function becomes increasingly compromised:
- Decreased synthetic function: Defective synthesis of proteins – for eg, albumin, clotting factors which

leads to coagulopathy and hypoalbuminemia.
- Impaired detoxification: Decreased HEPATIC METABOLISM leads to accumulation of toxic materials such as ammonia that causes hepatic encephalopathy.
- Altered metabolism: Disturbance in lipid, carbohydrate and protein metabolic process.

8. Complications of Cirrhosis
- Ascites: Development of changes in the abdominal cavity because of the increased pressure in the portal system and low albumin concentration in blood.
- Variceal bleeding: Varices in the oesophagus and stomach may develop, which can bleed heavily, threatening the patient's life.
- Hepatic encephalopathy: Neurological effects caused by toxins which include ammonia that tends to build up in the body.

- Hepatorenal syndrome: Liver failure complication that leads to other organs dysfunctioning, in this case, the kidneys.

9. Regenerative Nodules: In response to ongoing injury and fibrosis, the liver attempts to regenerate:
- Nodular regeneration: The liver in question develops nodules which are composed of regenerating hepatocytes and are enclosed by fibrous septa.
- These nodules are pathognomonic lesions and impair the normal architecture of the liver and aggravate the portal hypertension.

RISK FACTORS

1. Chronic Alcohol Consumption: Alcohol is the number one cause of liver cirrhosis, this being especially true due to binge and chronic drinking. Alcohol leads to liver cell inflammation, fat accumulation in liver cells, and over a number of years, cirrhosis of the liver.

2. Viral Hepatitis: Hepatitis B and C viruses have been known to cause cirrhosis at a global level. Whereas acute hepatitis B and C infections are typically resolved by the immune system, chronic cases of hepatitis B or C result in continued liver inflammation and scarring, which leads to cirrhosis.

3.Non Alcoholic Fatty Liver Disease (NAFLD): Obesity, Type 2 Diabetes mellitus, and metabolic syndrome are considered the common risk factors for NAFLD, which is taking the place of other liver diseases as the primary cirrhosis cause. This causes steatosis which when worsened by insulin resistance brings about Non-Alcoholic Steato hepatitis (NASH) that can result into cirrhosis.

4. Autoimmune Hepatitis: In autoimmune hepatitis the immune system is active against liver cells, and this results to inflammation and continuous damage to the liver cells. Consequently it can cause cirrhosis in case no treatment and intervention is taken.

5. Genetic Disorders: Certain inherited conditions increase the risk of liver cirrhosis, including:
- Hemochromatosis: Accumulation of iron in the human body especially in the liver.
- Wilson's Disease: Copper toxicity: this means an accumulation of copper in parts of the body, especially the liver, that has gone too high.

6. Biliary Diseases: Any pathologies that involve the bile duct include primary biliary cholangitis or PBC and primary sclerosing cholangitis or PSC, of which all result in inflammation and scarring of the bile duct leading to cirrhosis.

7. Chronic drug use and exposure to toxins: Some medicines for a long duration, including methotrexate, isoniazid, or environmental pollutants such as chemicals and hepato toxics, cause injury to the liver and make cirrhosis more probably.

8. Other Factors
- **Infections:** Some causes are: Chronic parasitic such as schistosomiasis may cause liver disease, cirrhosis included.

- **Non-alcoholic steatohepatitis (NASH):** Stages: Development of NAFLD to NASH leads to the risk of cirrhotic liver disease.

CLINICAL FEATURES
Early Clinical Features

In the early stages, cirrhosis may be asymptomatic or present with mild symptoms such as:
- **Fatigue** refers to the state of overall tiredness and low energy in an individual or a group.
- **Weakness**: Skeletal muscles become wasted and strength is decreased.
- **Loss of Appetite:** Disinterest towards eating
- **Nausea:** The sensation which may include feeling sick or vomiting.
- **Weight Loss:** Nutrition unrelated weight losing.
- **Itching (Pruritus**): This is because bile salts settle on the skin layers hence the greasy texture.

Late Clinical Features

As the disease progresses, more pronounced and serious symptoms develop, including:

- **Jaundice:** JCHOD: Jaundice characterized by the development of yellow pigmentation of the skin and sclera as a result of elevated bilirubin levels.
- **Edema:** Syndrome, peripheral edema meaning swelling in the legs and ankles due to accumulation of fluids.
- **Ascites:** Build up of fluid within the abdominal compartment which will make the belly look bigger.
- **Easy Bruising and Bleeding:** Because of a coagulation disorder called haemophilia and they also suffer from thrombocytopenia a disorder in which the body does not produce enough platelets in the blood.
- **Spider Angiomas:** Capillaries – small vessels that are clearly visible in skin, that weblike.
- **Palmar Erythema:** Although some signs such as redness of the palms are easier to identify, the condition of the skin may not be as reliable as

other signs, such as the degree of sweating.
- **Gynecomastia:** Gynaecomastia, refers to the condition whereby male breast tissue grows to become abnormally large.

DIAGNOSIS

Diagnosing liver cirrhosis involves a combination of medical history, physical examination, blood tests, imaging studies, and sometimes a liver biopsy:

1.Medical History and Physical Exam: In preparatory sessions, the doctor will sit down with you to understand medical history and resultant risks and signs. They will also assess your physical condition to look for features that may dignify cirrhosis for instance enlarged liver and spleen, yellow skin, and swelling.

2.Blood Tests: , the liver function tests like the international units for the liver enzymes of ALT, AST, and bilirubin will help determine the degree of liver injury. The extra tests may assess clotting abilities, the functioning of the kidneys or rule out any hepatitis infections.

3.Imaging Studies: Liver irregularities being a significant factor can be diagnosed using ultrasound method according to the specialist. Invasive biopsy procedures can be complemented with CT scans, MRI, or even elastography (FibroScan) to achieve better visualization and assess the liver elasticity.

4.Liver Biopsy: A biopsy of the liver may be taken where a small piece of the liver tissue is taken for microscopic examination to confirm the disease and the approximate degree of its advancement.

MANAGEMENT

Treatment of Liver Cirrhosis

The approach to treating liver cirrhosis involves the reduction of symptoms and signs, prevention of complication and treatment of the cause of the disease. Here are some key aspects of treatment:

1. Lifestyle changes

- **Alcohol Elimination:** If alcohol is cause of cirrhosis then alcohol elimination is a highly mandatory move.
- **Healthy Diet:** One's diet should include low quantities of salt since this assists in minimizing the level of fluids in the body. Hepatic encephalopathy could be a reason that needs alteration of protein consumption.
- **Weight Management:** NAFLD can be treated by weight loss which will be enhancing the health of the liver.

2. Medications:
- **Antiviral Medications:** For hepatitis B and C there are medications that can effectively manage the disease and stop further harm to the liver.
- **Medications to Control Symptoms:** Loosening of fluids may also be achieved by diuretics. It is also on Lactulose which may be used in managing hepatic encephalopathy.
- **Medications to Lower Portal Hypertension:** Beta blockers are useful to decrease the probability of having variceal bleeding.

3. Managing Complications:
- **Endoscopic Treatments:** Sharing of varix through band ligature or sclerotherapy can be helpful in controlling the bleeding from varix.
- **Paracentesis:** This operation entails the draining of fluid that accumulates in the abdomen particularly where ascitis is severe.

- **Antibiotics:** For management or prophylaxis of infections like spontaneous bacterial peritonitis.

4. Liver Transplant: In case the liver is extensively damaged, the only cure that can be offered to the patient is a liver transplant. This entails transplanting the liver of a healthy person for the diseased liver of the patient.

PREVENTING LIVER CIRRHOSIS
Preventing liver cirrhosis involves addressing the underlying causes and making lifestyle changes to protect liver health:
- **Limit Alcohol Consumption:** Alcohol should be limited or avoided so as to stop the alcohol from causing harm to the liver.
- **Maintain a Healthy Weight:** These have essentially confirmed that attainment of normal body weight through a healthy and well-portioned

diet and regular physical activity is the best preventative measure that can be taken against NAFLD accompanied by cirrhosis.
- **Get Vaccinated:** Hepatitis A and B can be vaccinated to eliminate chances of acquiring viral hepatits.
- **Avoid Risky Behaviors**: Measures like safe sex and not sharing needles should help lower the rate of hepatitis infection.
- **Regular Check-Ups:** Regular medical check-ups and screenings can help detect liver problems early and manage chronic conditions.

7-DAY DIET PLAN FOR LIVER CIRRHOSIS

DAY	BREAKFAST	LUNCH	DINNER
DAY 1	Scrambled eggs with spinach,	Turkey and avocado wrap with	Stir-fried tofu with vegetables

	whole grain toast	whole grain tortilla, side salad	and brown rice
DAY 2	Oatmeal with berries, a banana, herbal tea	Grilled chicken salad with mixed greens and vinaigrette, quinoa	Baked salmon, steamed broccoli, sweet potato
DAY 3	Smoothie with spinach, banana, and almond milk	Lentil soup, mixed greens salad with olive oil and lemon	Baked chicken breast, green beans, mashed potatoes
DAY 4	Whole grain pancakes with fresh fruit, herbal tea	Chickpea and vegetable stew, brown rice	Baked cod, asparagus, quinoa
DAY 5	Whole grain cereal with almond milk, berries	Grilled fish tacos with corn tortillas, cabbage slaw	Vegetable stir-fry with tofu and quinoa
DAY 6	Smoothie with kale,	Quinoa salad with	Grilled shrimp,

	berries, and flaxseed	black beans, corn, and tomatoes	mixed vegetables, brown rice
DAY 7	Avocado toast on whole grain bread, herbal tea	Chicken and vegetable skewers, quinoa	Baked turkey meatballs, steamed carrots, wild rice

PROGNOSIS

Liver cirrhosis can be referred to as the irreversible and continuous pathological process that results in the destruction of the hepatic parenchyma and formation of fibrous tissue. In terms of predicting the further development, the assessment of the prospects depends on the stage of liver cirrhosis, the cause of the disease, and the outcomes of the treatments applied. At this stage, the major cause of cirrhosis should be eliminated avoiding alcohol, managing the conditions like hepatitis, and having a healthy diet to slow the pace of the disease and enhance the quality of life. Sometimes medications may be administered in order to control the symptoms as well as the complications that are bound to occur. Several complications develop as an unstoppable progression to cirrhotic liver disease and consists of liver failure, variceal bleeding, formation of an ascites, hepatic encephalopathy, and hepatic malignancy. Thus, in some cases, the only treatment is a liver transplant in the late stages of the disease.

Medical care especially timely diagnosis is very important to slow the progression of cirrhosis and increase the life duration. A ruling out of symptoms and a compliance with medical regimens go a long way in improving the prognosis.

CHAPTER 3

HEMOCHROMATOSIS

Hemochromatosis can also be defined as an iron overload condition. The body has ways of controlling how much iron it absorbs from the food it ingests, but in individuals with the disease, this mechanism is impaired. In so doing, the body stores more iron than it requires from the diet and this extra iron accumulates in tissues and organs. In the long run, such damage occurs, and these organs lose their functionality as an outcome.

TYPES OF HEMOCHROMATOSIS

There are various forms of hemochromatosis, each with different causes and characteristics:

1. Hereditary Hemochromatosis (Type 1): This type is the most prevalent and is linked to the Hemochromatosis gene also abbreviated as HFE gene. It usually affects adults, male and females with symptoms developing in the 3rd, 4th and 5th decades for male and post-menopausal for females.

2. Juvenile Hemochromatosis (Types 2A and 2B): This is a less frequent form provoked by the mutations of HJV (hemojuvelin) or HAMP (hepcidin) and occurs at the early age. The patient requires early and appropriate treatment because it can results to severe iron overload and complications at a young age.

3.Neonatal Hemochromatosis: This is an extremely rare form and the infants develop symptoms at birth or within the first few days of life and the liver is significantly affected.

4.Secondary Hemochromatosis: It is not hereditary, though it can develop due to another disorder or a factor that contributes to the buildup of iron levels in the blood such as multiple blood transfusions, some forms of anemia, or chronic liver disease.

EPIDEMIOLOGY

1. Prevalence: Hereditary haemochromatosis is estimated to have a prevalence of between one in 200 and one in 500 depending on the population studied most commonly in individuals of Northern European origin. The carrier rate (heterozygotes) is higher and empowering carrier rate ranging one out of eight to one out of ten of this particular population.

2. Genetic Basis: Over 90% of the cases can be associated with the pathological mutations within the HFE gene, namely C282Y and H63D. The C282Y mutation is particularly linked to clinical hemochromatosis, and C282Y homozygosity has the strongest correlation with phenotypic expression of the disease.

3. Age and Gender: Ideally, symptoms emerge in male patients aged forty to sixty years and in female patients who are postmenopausal because iron builds up at a slower pace in women because of their monthly periods.

4. Geographical Distribution: It is also more common in people of Northern European origin and its occurrence is low in African and Asian Indians, and Hispanic populations. I haemochromatosis, early diagnosis and treatment and possible through phlebotomy reduced the severity of the symptoms of the disease and enhanced the quality of individuals life.

CAUSES AND RISK FACTORS

Hereditary hemochromatosis is an inherited disorder that results from genetic flaws in genes. Identifying the cause of hereditary haemochromatosis, the most frequent mutation is the HFE gene with C282Y and H63D variants. People who receive two mutant genes one from their mother and the other from the father are at a greater chance of contracting the disease. Family History: Other risk factors include:

1.Family history of hemochromatosis: people with a first-degree relative with the condition is at a higher risk.

2.Ethnicity: They discovered that the HFE gene mutations were more common in people with Northern European origins.

3.Gender: Males seem to develop symptoms early than females, probably due to regular Iron loss through menstruation and pregnancy.

CLINICAL FEATURES OF HEMOCHROMATOSIS

1.General Symptoms: Fatigue and weakness Joint pain, particularly in the hands and knees weight loss.

2. Skin: Bronze or gray skin pigmentation (often referred to as "bronzing")

3. Liver: Hepatomegaly (enlarged liver),liver cirrhosis,liver cancer (hepatocellular carcinoma).

4. Endocrine: Diabetes mellitus (often referred to as "bronze diabetes" due to skin pigmentation),hypogonadism (leading to symptoms such as loss of libido, impotence, amenorrhea) and hypothyroidism.

5. Cardiovascular: Cardiomyopathy (leading to heart failure),arrhythmias (irregular heartbeats).

6. Joints: Arthralgia (joint pain),arthritis particularly in the hands (e.g., second and third metacarpophalangeal joints).

7. Pancreas: Diabetes mellitus due to iron deposition in the pancreas.

8. Reproductive: Testicular atrophy in men and menstrual irregularities in women.

9. CNS and Other Organs: Memory loss, cognitive difficulties and Increased susceptibility to certain infections due to iron's effect on the immune system.

DIAGNOSIS OF HEMOCHROMATOSIS

It is important that the condition should be diagnosed at a very early stage to avoid the damaging of organs. The diagnostic process typically involves:

1. Medical History and Physical Exam: The doctor will then want to know about the patient's medical history and that of other family members, then they will conduct a physical examination for symptoms of iron overload.

2. Blood Tests:
- **Serum Ferritin:** C, measures the concentration of stored iron in the

human body. With higher level indications of iron overload.

- **Transferrin Saturation:** Estimates the number of transferrin-sites occupied by iron, transferrin is a protein which transports iron in blood. High levels suggest hemochromatosis.

- **Liver Function Tests:** To diagnose liver diseases or illnesses or to check the general health of a person's liver.

3. Genetic Testing: To ascertain that HFE gene mutations are present. This is perhaps useful if there has been a hereditary line to the disease within the family of the patient.

4. Liver Biopsy: Sometimes, a biopsy may be carried out in order to determine the severity of liver injury and/or the amount of iron deposited in it.

5. MRI and Imaging Studies: It is also agreed that MRI can be done to determine the level of iron in liver and other organs.

MANAGEMENT OF HEMOCHROMATOSIS

LIVING WITH HEMOCHROMATOSIS
Control of the condition and maintaining certain changes to avoid development of other related complications. Here are some tips:

1. Medical Check-Ups: Ensure you honor doctor appointments often for your iron levels and organ checks, or any other complications arising from the injury.

2. Healthy Diet: A balanced diet should be consumed together with extra precaution taken especially on meals that are rich in iron. Abstain from alcohol that can worsen the liver condition even further.

3. Exercise: It is thus clear that the process of undergoing exercising aids in enhancing the general health of a human being.

4. Educate Yourself: The more a patient knows about their particular type of hemochromatosis the better prepared they are for news treatments and new research in their type of haemochromatosis.

5.**Support Groups:** It is essential to find and interact with individuals having hemochromatosis to see how they cope with the condition and get adequate information.

TREATMENT

The primary goal of treatment is to remove excess iron from the body and prevent further accumulation. The main treatments include:

1. Phlebotomy: This is the most common and effective treatment for hereditary hemochromatosis. It involves regularly removing blood (similar to donating blood) to reduce iron levels. Initially, this may be done weekly until iron levels normalize, followed by maintenance phlebotomies every few months.

2. Chelation Therapy: For patients who cannot undergo phlebotomy (e.g., those with anemia or heart problems), medications called iron chelators can be used. These drugs bind to iron and help remove it from the body through urine or feces.

3. Monitoring and Managing Complications: Regular follow-up appointments are crucial to monitor iron levels and manage any complications, such as liver disease, diabetes, or heart problems.

4. Dietary Changes: While diet alone cannot manage iron overload, certain dietary adjustments can help:

- **Avoid Iron Supplements and Multivitamins**: Unless prescribed by a doctor.
- **Limit Vitamin C Intake**: As it can increase iron absorption.

7-DAY DIET PLAN FOR A PATIENT WITH HEMOCHROMATOSIS

DAY	BREAKFAST	LUNCH	DINNER
DAY 1	Oatmeal with almond milk, berries, herbal tea and Apple slices with almond	Grilled chicken salad with mixed greens, vinaigrette	Baked salmon, steamed broccoli, brown rice

DAY 2	Scrambled eggs with spinach, whole grain toast	Turkey and avocado wrap with whole grain tortilla, side salad	Stir-fried tofu with vegetables and quinoa
DAY 3	Smoothie with kale, banana, almond milk	Lentil soup, mixed greens salad with olive oil	Baked chicken breast, green beans, quinoa
DAY 4	Whole grain cereal with almond milk, berries	Quinoa and vegetable salad with olive oil and lemon Greek yogurt and Greek yogurt with fruit	Vegetable stir-fry with tofu and brown rice
DAY 5	Whole grain pancakes with fresh fruit, herbal tea	Chickpea and vegetable stew, brown rice	Baked turkey meatballs, steamed carrots, wild rice
DAY 6	Avocado toast on whole grain	Chicken and vegetable	Baked turkey meatballs,

54

	bread, herbal tea	skewers, quinoa	steamed carrots, wild rice
DAY 7	Smoothie with spinach, berries, and flaxseedwith Handful of pistachios	Quinoa salad with black beans, corn, and tomatoes	Grilled shrimp, mixed vegetables, brown rice Apple slices with almond butter

NOTES:

Protein: Give special attention to lean protein sources including turkey, chicken, fish, and beans and tofu from plants.

Iron: Steer clear of meals enriched with iron and consume less red meat. When feasible, get your protein from plant-based sources.

Vitamin C: To improve the absorption of iron, limit the amount of foods high in vitamin C that you eat between meals.

Dairy: Add dairy products to your diet as

they may help prevent the absorption of iron.

Whole Grains: Avoid whole grains fortified with iron, but choose whole grains instead of processed grains.

Always get advice from a dietitian or healthcare professional to make sure the meal plan satisfies the unique requirements and limitations of the hemochromatosis patient.

PROGNOSIS

Those who with hemochromatosis can live normal, healthy lives provided they receive early diagnosis and appropriate care. Early therapy initiation is crucial to prevent major organ damage. Most problems may be avoided and a high quality of life can be maintained with routine monitoring and care.

CHAPTER 4

HEPATITIS B

Hepatitis B is an infective disease of the liver caused by Hepatitis B virus. It comes from hepatitis B virus (HBV). HBV is transmitted through blood and other bodily fluids contaminated with the virus. Depending on the particular circumstances, hepatitis B infection can be acute or chronic. Conversely, acute hepatitis B lasts a short duration and does not cause severe complications, though chronic hepatitis B is known to cause conditions such as cirrhosis and liver cancer. Hepatitis B is one illness that can be prevented through vaccination since there is a vaccine that does this.

EPIDEMIOLOGY

As of 2019, 296 million people worldwide were chronically infected with hepatitis B virus (HBV). Hepatitis B is a very common infectious disease.

1. Regional differences exist in the prevalence of hepatitis B: Regions with high prevalence: The Pacific Islands, East Asia, and Sub-Saharan Africa have the greatest rates of hepatitis B infection. In these regions, the virus is frequently passed from mother to child at birth or during early infancy from one individual to another.

2. Regions with intermediate prevalence: South Asia, the Middle East, and Eastern Europe exhibit intermediate rates of persistent HBV infection.

3. Low-prevalence regions: Because of more effective immunization campaigns as well as improved screening and treatment options, the prevalence rates are lower in North America, Western Europe, and Australia.

PATHOPHYSIOLOGY

The pathophysiology of hepatitis B involves complex interactions between the virus and the host's immune system. Here is an overview of the key steps in the disease process:

1. Viral Entry and Replication: HBV enters the body and infects liver cells (hepatocytes). The virus's DNA is transported to the cell nucleus, where it is converted into covalently closed circular DNA (cccDNA), serving as a template for viral replication. The virus replicates using the host cell machinery to produce new viral particles.

2. Immune Response: The body's immune response to HBV infection determines the clinical outcome. In acute infection, a strong, multi-faceted immune response usually clears the virus, resulting in resolution. In chronic infection, an inadequate immune response allows the virus to persist, leading to ongoing liver inflammation and damage.

3. Liver Damage: The liver damage in hepatitis B is primarily immune-mediated. Cytotoxic T cells attack infected hepatocytes, causing cell death and inflammation. Over time, chronic inflammation can lead to fibrosis, cirrhosis, and an increased risk of liver cancer.

RISK FACTORS

Hepatitis B risk is increased by a number of factors:

1. Unprotected Sex: The risk of transmission is increased when an infected person engages in unprotected sex.

2. Perinatal Transmission: There is a significant chance that newborns of infected mothers will contract hepatitis B.

3. Blood Transfusions and Organ Transplants: The virus can be spread by receiving blood products or organs from an infected donor.

4. Needle Sharing: Sharing syringes or needles poses a serious risk, particularly for intravenous drug users.

5. Healthcare Exposure: The possibility of coming into contact with bodily fluids and blood that are infectious puts healthcare workers at risk.

6. Close contact: Living in close proximity to someone who suffers from chronic hepatitis B increases the chance of infection, especially in areas where the disease is endemic.

7. Travel: There is a higher chance of contracting hepatitis B when visiting areas with a high incidence of the infection.

Depending on whether the infection is acute or chronic, there are different ways that hepatitis B can manifest:

CLINICAL FEATURES
Acute Hepatitis B:
- **Asymptomatic:** Many people with acute hepatitis B are asymptomatic, especially children.

- **Symptomatic:** When symptoms do appear, they may include fatigue, loss of appetite, nausea, vomiting, abdominal pain, dark urine, pale stools, and jaundice (yellowing of the skin and eyes).

Chronic Hepatitis B:
- **Asymptomatic Phase:** Asymptomatic Hepatitis B can remain asymptomatic for many years.

- **Symptomatic Phase:** When symptoms of chronic hepatitis B manifest, they may include jaundice, abdominal pain, and joint pain. Over time, chronic hepatitis B can cause cirrhosis and liver failure, with symptoms like ascites (fluid accumulation in the abdomen), easy bruising, and bleeding.

DIAGNOSIS

Diagnosing hepatitis B involves a combination of blood tests and imaging studies:

1.Serologic Tests: These tests detect specific antigens and antibodies related to HBV infection:

- HBsAg (Hepatitis B surface antigen): Indicates active HBV infection.
- Anti-HBs (Hepatitis B surface antibody): Indicates immunity to HBV,

either from past infection or vaccination.
- Anti-HBc (Hepatitis B core antibody): Indicates previous or ongoing infection.
- HBeAg (Hepatitis B e antigen): Indicates active viral replication and high infectivity.
- Anti-HBe (Hepatitis B e antibody): Indicates a lower level of viral replication.

2. HBV DNA Testing: Measures the amount of viral DNA in the blood, indicating the level of viral replication.

3. Liver Function Tests: Assess the extent of liver damage and inflammation.

4. Imaging Studies: Ultrasound, CT scans, and MRI can evaluate liver damage and detect complications like cirrhosis or liver cancer.

5. Liver Biopsy: In some cases, a liver biopsy may be performed to assess the extent of liver damage and fibrosis.

MANAGEMENT

The management of hepatitis B depends on the phase of the infection (acute or chronic) and the patient's overall health:

Acute Hepatitis B:

- **Supportive Care:** Most cases of acute hepatitis B do not require specific antiviral treatment. Supportive care, including rest, adequate nutrition, and hydration, is usually sufficient.
- **Monitoring:** Patients should be monitored for signs of chronic infection.

Chronic Hepatitis B:

- **Antiviral Medications:** Several antiviral drugs are available to treat chronic hepatitis B, including:
    - **Nucleos(t)ide Analogues**: Such as tenofovir, entecavir, and lamivudine, which inhibit viral replication.
    - **Pegylated Interferon:** Boosts the immune response against the virus

- **Monitoring and Surveillance:** Regular monitoring of liver function, HBV DNA levels, and screening for liver cancer are essential.

- **Liver Transplant:** In cases of severe liver damage or liver failure, a liver transplant may be necessary.

- **Lifestyle Modifications:** Patients should avoid alcohol and hepatotoxic medications and maintain a healthy diet and weight.

FOODS FOR HEPATITIS PATIENTS

Here is a table outlining foods that a hepatitis B patient should consume and those they should avoid to support liver health and overall well-being.

Recommended Foods	Foods to Avoid
Lean Proteins: chicken, turkey, fish, tofu, beans	High-Fat Meats: fatty cuts of beef, pork, lamb
Whole Grains: brown rice, quinoa, whole wheat bread, oats	Refined Carbs: white bread, pastries, sugary cereals
Fruits: apples, berries, oranges, pears	Sugary Foods: candy, sweets, desserts
Vegetables: leafy greens, broccoli, carrots, bell peppers	Fried Foods: fried chicken, french fries, potato chips
Healthy Fats: olive oil, avocados, nuts, seeds	Trans Fats: margarine, processed snacks
Low-Fat Dairy: skim milk, yogurt, cheese	Full-Fat Dairy: whole milk, cream, full-fat cheese
Hydration: water, herbal teas	Alcohol: beer, wine, spirits

Legumes: lentils, chickpeas, black beans	High-Sodium Foods: canned soups, processed meats, salty snacks
Herbs and Spices: turmeric, garlic, ginger	High-Sugar Drinks: soda, fruit juices with added sugar
Omega-3 Rich Foods: salmon, flaxseeds, walnuts	Processed Foods: ready meals, packaged snacks

NOTE

- **Protein:** Choose foods that have lean proteins as this will help in the functioning of the liver without putting extra work to the liver to digest fats.

- **Whole Grains:** These give fiber and necessary nutrients which are not accompanied by surges in blood sugar levels as observed in refined grains.

- **Fruits and Vegetables:** Packed in antioxidants, vitamins, and minerals,

- **Progressive Disease:** Others may develop progressive liver disease, including cirrhosis, liver failure, and hepatocellular carcinoma.
- **Survival:** With appropriate management and regular monitoring, many people with chronic hepatitis B can live long, healthy lives. However, the risk of liver-related complications remains.

CHAPTER 5

HEPATITIS C

Hepatitis C is a viral infection that primarily affects the liver, causing inflammation and potentially leading to severe liver damage. It is caused by the hepatitis C virus (HCV) and is one of the most common causes of chronic liver disease worldwide. Hepatitis C can be acute or chronic, with the chronic form posing significant long-term health risks, including cirrhosis, liver failure, and hepatocellular carcinoma. This guide provides an in-depth look at hepatitis C, including its epidemiology, pathophysiology, risk factors, clinical features, diagnosis, management, and prognosis.

EPIDEMIOLOGY

Hepatitis C is a world wide problem with approximately 71 million carriers of the virus reported around the globe. According to some data, the rates of HCV are different and the higher level is traced in the countries of Central and East Asia, North Africa, and the Middle East. Epidemiologists estimate that in the USA there are around 2.4 million sufferers of chronic hepatitis C.

While as modern techniques of blood screening, safer medical, practices, improved hygiene, renal replacement therapy and better health management have collectively has significantly brought down the new cases of infection in many developed countries. Nevertheless, hepatitis C is still a significant public health issue because of its capability to cause chronic hepatitis, the asymptomatic course of its initial stage, and its spread through some specific risky practices.

PATHOPHYSIOLOGY

Hepatitis C is an RNA virus that affects the liver mainly the hepatocytes cells in the liver. Once the HCV virus has penetrated the blood stream immediately begins to penetrate and invade the liver cells and then proceeds to use the cells replicating machinery. The immune system also targets infected liver cells in an attempt to destroy the virus and in the process the liver is damaged.

HCV is known to infect most people quickly and is capable of mutating and thus, avoiding the body's immune response most of the time. Thus, chronic hepatitis C is characterized by constant inflammation of the liver which over time may result in fibrosis and cirrhosis. They also get resolved by themselves or progress to chronic HCV infection that can cause cirrhosis or hepatocellular carcinoma in certain circumstances.

- Most people with acute hepatitis C are asymptomatic or have mild, nonspecific symptoms.
- When symptoms occur, they may include fatigue, fever, nausea, vomiting, abdominal pain, dark urine, clay-colored stools, and jaundice.

- Acute infection can spontaneously clear in some individuals, particularly those with a strong immune response.

2. Chronic Hepatitis C:

- Many individuals with chronic hepatitis C remain asymptomatic for years, even decades.

- Symptoms, when present, can include persistent fatigue, joint pain, itchy skin, muscle aches, and cognitive issues such as brain fog.

- As the disease progresses, signs of liver damage such as jaundice, ascites (fluid buildup in the abdomen), easy bruising, and bleeding may develop.

DIAGNOSIS

The diagnosis of hepatitis C involves several steps:

1. **Serologic Tests**:
    - **Anti-HCV Antibody Test**: This test detects antibodies to HCV, indicating past or present infection.
    - **HCV RNA Test**: Confirms active infection by detecting the presence of viral RNA in the blood.
2. **Genotyping**: Determining the specific genotype of HCV is important for treatment planning, as different

genotypes respond differently to antiviral therapies.

3. **Liver Function Tests:** Assess liver health and function, including levels of ALT, AST, bilirubin, and alkaline phosphatase.

4. **Liver Biopsy and Imaging:** In some cases, a liver biopsy or imaging studies such as transient elastography (FibroScan) or MRI may be performed to assess the extent of liver damage and fibrosis.

MANAGEMENT

The management of hepatitis C has evolved significantly with the development of direct-acting antivirals (DAAs), which offer high cure rates with shorter treatment durations and fewer side effects compared to older therapies.

1.Antiviral Therapy:

- Direct-Acting Antivirals (DAAs): DAAs target specific steps in the HCV life cycle, effectively eradicating the virus in most patients. Treatment regimens typically last 8 to 12 weeks and vary based on HCV genotype, liver function, and prior treatment history.
- Interferon and Ribavirin: These older treatments are now rarely used due to their lower efficacy and higher side effect profiles compared to DAAs.

2. Monitoring and Supportive Care:

- Regular monitoring of liver function and viral load during and after treatment.
- Lifestyle modifications such as avoiding alcohol, maintaining a healthy diet, and managing comorbid conditions like diabetes and obesity.

3. Liver Transplantation:

In cases of advanced liver disease or liver cancer, liver transplantation may be necessary. Post-transplant patients require antiviral treatment to prevent HCV recurrence in the new liver.

FOOD FOR HEPATITIS C

The foods that a patient with hepatitis C should eat and should not eat are included in this table. The goal of this is to promote general health and liver wellness.

Foods to Include	Foods to Avoid
Lean Proteins: - Chicken, turkey, fish, tofu, beans	Alcohol: - All forms (beer, wine, spirits)
Whole Grains:- Brown rice, whole wheat bread, quinoa, oats	High-Fat Foods:- Fried foods, fast food, high-fat dairy products
Fruits and Vegetables:- Leafy greens, berries, citrus fruits, carrots, broccoli	Processed Foods:- Packaged snacks, processed meats, sugary cereals

Healthy Fats:- Avocado, nuts, seeds, olive oil	High-Sodium Foods:- Canned soups, processed meats, salty snacks
Dairy:- Low-fat or fat-free yogurt, milk, cheese	Sugary Foods:- Sugary drinks, desserts, candies
Hydration:- Water, herbal teas	Raw or Undercooked Foods:- Sushi, raw shellfish, undercooked meats
High-Fiber Foods:- Whole fruits, vegetables, legumes, whole grains	Trans Fats:- Margarine, packaged baked goods
Nutrient-Rich Foods:- Eggs, lean meat, fish, legumes	Red and Processed Meats: - Bacon, sausage, hot dogs
Antioxidant-Rich Foods:- Blueberries, spinach, nuts	Caffeine:- Limit intake of coffee and caffeinated drinks

PROGNOSIS

The prognosis for hepatitis C varies depending on whether the infection is acute or chronic and the presence of complications:The prognosis for hepatitis B varies depending on whether the infection is acute or chronic and the presence of complications:

Acute Hepatitis C:

- **Resolution:** The majority of the adult patients with acute Hepatitis C regain full health, and they have immune status for life.

- **Chronic Infection:** In some cases, around 5-10% of adults with acute hepatitis B develop chronic infection while nearly 90% of infants, and one in four to one in ten children get chronic infection.

Chronic Hepatitis C:

- **Stable Disease:** Chronic hepatitis C disease flows that some people even with the above symptoms have normal liver enzymes and are not affected.

- **Progressive Disease:** Some people may end up with other progressive liver disease such as cirrhosis liver failure and hepatocellular carcinoma.

- **Survival:** As with many chronic conditions if properly cared for and closely monitored an individual with hepatitis C can live a normal satisfactory length of life. But the prospects of liver complication related mishap persists and in fact are a known tangible possibility.

CHAPTER 6

PRIMARY BILIARY CHOLANGITIS (PBC)

Primary biliary cholangitis (PBC), earlier referred to as primary biliary cirrhosis, is a corrosive liver disease where the medium-sized mixed ducts inside the liver are gradually destroyed by inflammation. This destruction therefore comes with a dysfunction of bile flow commonly referred to as cholestasis in which bile stagnate in the liver causing liver injury. Long-term consequence of the described processes includes fibrosis, cirrhosis, and liver failure. Knowledge of PBC is necessary for early diagnosis and treatment that will help enhance the quality of life of persons with the illness.

EPIDEMIOLOGY

1.Prevalence:

- PBC is considered a rare disease with varying prevalence worldwide.
- The prevalence ranges from 1.91 to 40.2 per 100,000 individuals, depending on the region and population studied.

2. Incidence:
- Incidence rates vary widely but generally range from 0.33 to 5.8 per 100,000 person-years.
- Higher incidence rates are reported in Europe and North America compared to Asia.

3. Gender Distribution:
- PBC predominantly affects women, with a female-to-male ratio of about 9:1.

- This gender disparity is a hallmark of the disease and suggests a possible hormonal or genetic influence.

4. Age of Onset:
- The typical age of onset is between 40 and 60 years.
- It is rare in individuals under 25 years old.

5. Geographical Variation:
- Higher prevalence and incidence rates are reported in Northern Europe and North America.
- Lower rates are observed in Asian countries, although increasing trends have been noted in some regions.

6. Risk Factors:
- Genetic predisposition plays a significant role, with family members of affected individuals having a higher risk.
- Environmental factors, such as infections and exposure to certain chemicals, are also thought to contribute.

- Smoking, hormone replacement therapy, and urinary tract infections have been implicated as potential risk factors.

7. **Ethnic Differences:**
   - PBC is more common in Caucasians compared to other ethnic groups.
   - Studies indicate lower prevalence in African American and Hispanic populations.

PATHOPHYSIOLOGY

The actual aetiology of PBC is not well described, however, most practitioners agree that the illness is auto-immune in nature. Autoimmune disorder affects the small bile ducts in the liver in this situation, where the body's immune system is at work destroying it gradually. Several factors contribute to the pathogenesis of PBC:

1. Family History: Family history is important in designing treatment of PBC because people with family history of PBC are vulnerable to developing it. It has also been observed that some of the allelic variants of the DNA sequence from the HLA complex are higher in patients with the type of this disease; particularly the HLA-DRB1*08.

2. Environmental Triggers: These infections and other burdens such as exposure to chemical and smoking are cited to have played key roles in activating the autoimmune gene amongst the susceptible members.

3. Immune System Dysregulation: In the immune system, autoantibodies are produced in which antimitochondrial antibodies are typical, and they attack the lining of the ducts in the bile. This autoimmune process results in Cholestasis, fibrosis and can result to complete obliteration of the bile ducts.

4. Cholestasis: The gradual degeneration of the amphibian's bile ducts leads to cholestasis, which is the congesting of the liver with bile. On continuing the process the liver becomes damaged it becomes inflamed and fibrosis sets in.

RISK FACTORS

Several factors increase the risk of developing PBC:

1. Gender: Women are at a significantly higher risk than men, with approximately 90% of PBC cases occurring in females.

2. Age: PBC typically affects individuals between the ages of 40 and 60.

3. Genetics: A family history of PBC or other autoimmune diseases increases the risk, suggesting a genetic predisposition.

4. Environmental Factors: Exposure to certain chemicals, infections, and smoking have been associated with an increased risk of PBC.

5. Other Autoimmune Diseases: PBC is often associated with other autoimmune conditions, such as Sjögren's syndrome, autoimmune thyroid disease, and rheumatoid arthritis.

CLINICAL FEATURES

Patient with PBC may present in numerous ways, and diagnosis can be highly complicated although still important since primary biliary cirrhosis is a fatal ailment. There are patients without any clinical symptoms and are discovered during some blood tests or other occasional investigations while others have vague or even severe clinical manifestations. Common clinical features include:

1. Fatigue: Fatigue is one of the most predominant and long-standing symptoms of PBC and may cause a serious diminution of the patient's quality of life.

2. Pruritus (Itching): Pruritus, a general itching mainly at night, is also commonly seen and may be severe.

3. Jaundice: In its more serious and developed forms, unveiling of skin and sclerae is observed as a result of rising of bilirubin content.

4. Hepatomegaly: Hepatomegaly is a frequent finding and may be evaluated during the evaluation of the subject.

5. Xanthomas and Xanthelasmas: These are cholestates that become yellowish on the skin often around the eyes usually called xanthelasmas or large nodules on elbows, knees palmar surface and sole referred to as xanthomas.

6. Dry Eyes and Mouth: Most people with PBC develop sicca syndrome – dry eyes and a dry mouth as the patient is associated with Sjogren's syndrome.

7. Bone and Joint Pain: It can cause osteopenia, osteoporosis or arthritis and the patient may develop joint pain and fragile bones.

DIAGNOSIS

The diagnosis of PBC involves a combination of clinical evaluation, laboratory tests, imaging studies, and sometimes liver biopsy. Key diagnostic steps include:

1. Medical History and Physical Examination: A thorough history and physical exam to assess symptoms, risk factors, and signs of liver disease.

2. Laboratory Tests:

- **Liver Function Tests (LFTs):** Elevated levels of alkaline phosphatase (ALP) and gamma-glutamyl transferase (GGT) are common in PBC.
- **Antimitochondrial Antibodies (AMAs):** The presence of AMAs in the blood is highly specific for PBC and found in about 95% of patients
- **Other Autoantibodies:** Testing for other autoantibodies, such as antinuclear antibodies (ANAs), may be performed.

3. **Imaging Studies:**
    - **Ultrasound:** To assess liver size, structure, and rule out other causes of liver disease.
    - **Magnetic Resonance Imaging (MRI) and Magnetic Resonance Cholangiopancreatography (MRCP):** To evaluate bile ducts and liver tissue in more detail.

4. Liver Biopsy: While not always necessary, a liver biopsy can confirm the diagnosis and assess the extent of liver damage and fibrosis.

MANAGEMENT

Management of PBC has its main objective of reducing the speed at which the disease progresses, relieve symptoms, and reduce the risk of associated complications. Treatment options include:

1. Ursodeoxycholic Acid (UDCA): UDCA is the initial medication of the first choice for the treatment of PBC. It aids the right flowing of bile, decrease inflammation of the liver and arrested the advancement of diseases. Generally, UDCA therapy yields better results for most patients, although there may be cases in which extra treatment is needed.

2. Obeticholic Acid (OCA): OCA is a recently developed agent, which in addition to UDCA or as a sole therapy for those non-UDCA responders. The way it operates is that it decreases the production of bile acids and increased the rate at which bile can move through the body.

3. Symptom Management:

- **Pruritus:** For itching you can use cholestyramine, rifampicin, naltrexone, and sertraline.
- **Fatigue:** It is possible for a person to minimise fatigue through modifying their lifestyle, exercising, as well as controlling other diseases.

4. Management of Complications:

- **Osteoporosis:** Beside bisphosphonates, calcium and vitamin

D are useful in controlling the process of bone density drop.
- **Hyperlipidemia:** Antilipidemics like statins can be taken Sometimes.
- **Dry Eyes and Mouth:** Sjogrens syndrome can be treated through the use of artificial tears and saliva, mobility and stimulant substances such as pilocarpine and cevimeline among others.

5. Liver Transplantation: In cases where liver failure has been realized, then one is likely to require a liver transplantation. PBC is presently among a short list of diseases that indicate the need for a liver transplant.

7 DAY DIETARY PLAN FOR A PATIENT WITH PBC

Here's a 7-day dietary plan for a patient with primary biliary cholangitis (PBC), focusing on balanced nutrition to support liver health.

This plan includes low-fat, high-fiber foods, and ensures adequate intake of vitamins and minerals.

Day	Breakfast	Lunch	Dinner
Monday	Oatmeal with berries and a splash of almond milk	Grilled chicken salad with olive oil dressing, whole grain bread	Baked salmon, quinoa, steamed broccoli
Tuesday	Scrambled eggs with spinach and a slice of whole grain toast	Lentil soup, mixed green salad and whole grain crackers	Turkey breast, sweet potato, green beans
Wednesday	Greek yogurt with honey and a handful of nuts	Quinoa salad with chickpeas, cucumber, tomato, and feta cheese	Grilled chicken breast, brown rice, steamed carrots

Thursday	Smoothie with spinach, banana, and almond milk	Turkey sandwich on whole grain bread, side salad	Baked cod, mashed cauliflower, roasted Brussels sprouts
Friday	Whole grain toast with avocado and a boiled egg	Grilled chicken wrap with veggies and hummus	Baked tofu, wild rice, sautéed spinach
Saturday	Oatmeal with flaxseeds and a splash of almond milk	Baked salmon, barley, steamed asparagus	Lean beef stir-fry with broccoli, carrots, and brown rice
Sunday	Scrambled tofu with veggies and a slice of whole grain toast	Chicken and vegetable stir-fry with brown rice	Grilled shrimp, quinoa, sautéed green beans

PROGNOSIS

PBC has been also found to be of good prognosis especially when the disease is diagnosed early enough and gets treated. In many patients with PBC, the disease does not significantly limit the quality of life if the proper treatment is employed. It is a chronic disease, with the prognosis generally good in patients taking UDCA since most have a favourable outcome regarding liver complications. Hepatologist follow-up and evaluations should be conducted at standard time intervals for examination of symptoms, functioning of liver, and management of possible complications. For conditions of the last stage of the disease with cirrhosis and liver failure, transplantation offers an opportunity for salvage with relatively good long-term prognosis. Ideally, PBC should be diagnosed at an early stage consistent with the goal of early treatment, in order to enhance the quality of life and prognosis.

CHAPTER 7

PRIMARY SCLEROSING CHOLANGITIS (PSC)

Primary Sclerosing Cholangitis (PSC) is a non-detectable, cholestatic, slowly progressive liver disease that involves sclerosis and stricturing of the intrahepatic and extrahepatic bile ducts. These bile ducts which transport bile from the liver to the gallbladder and the small intestine become affected by fibrosis and thus blocked and there is a risk that the liver may be affected as well. As a matter of fact, at this given point in time, all of the causes of PSC have not been determined, and this disease presents a troubled picture regarding diagnosis and successful treatment. The following guide intends to offer an ample general outlook on the PSC: Epidemiology, etiology, risk quantifiers, manifestations, diagnosing, treatment, and prognosis.

EPIDEMIOLOGY

PSC is believed to be a rather limited condition, although it is present in different countries in differing measure. This is anticipated to be apparent in about seven to 15 cases per 1 million populace of the western folks. It is more commonly diagnosed in men than in women, with a male-to-female ratio of about 2:First of all: The disease mostly develops for people in the age range between 30 and 40 years, though it is not restricted to this age bracket. PSC is strongly connected with IBD, mainly ulcerative colitis, which is diagnosed in 70–80% of PSC patients. The epidemiology of PSC is on the rise, and this could probably be attributed to better diagnosis resulting from the enhanced awareness.

PATHOPHYSIOLOGY

The exact cause of PSC remains unknown, but it is believed to involve a combination of genetic, immunological, and environmental factors. The disease is characterized by chronic inflammation and fibrosis of the bile ducts, both intrahepatic (within the liver) and extrahepatic (outside the liver). This fibrosis leads to the formation of strictures, which can obstruct bile flow and cause bile to accumulate in the liver. The persistent inflammation and bile stasis eventually result in liver damage, fibrosis, and cirrhosis.

Several theories have been proposed to explain the pathogenesis of PSC:

1. Genetic Predisposition: Certain genetic factors may increase susceptibility to PSC. Studies have identified several genetic loci associated with an increased risk of PSC, including HLA haplotypes.

2. Immune-Mediated Mechanisms: PSC is thought to be an autoimmune disease, as evidenced by the presence of autoantibodies and the association with other autoimmune conditions, such as IBD. The immune system may mistakenly attack the bile ducts, leading to chronic inflammation and fibrosis.

3. Microbial Factors: Changes in the gut microbiome and bacterial translocation across the intestinal barrier may play a role in the development of PSC. This is supported by the strong association between PSC and IBD.

4. Environmental Triggers: Environmental factors, such as infections or toxins, may trigger or exacerbate PSC in genetically predisposed individuals.

RISK FACTORS

Several risk factors have been identified that may increase the likelihood of developing PSC:

1.Inflammatory Bowel Disease (IBD): The most significant risk factor for PSC is the presence of IBD, particularly ulcerative colitis. Crohn's disease is also associated with PSC but to a lesser extent.

2. Genetic Factors: A family history of PSC or other autoimmune diseases can increase the risk of developing PSC. Certain genetic markers, such as HLA-B8 and HLA-DR3, have been associated with PSC.

3. Male Gender: PSC is more common in men than in women.

4. Age: PSC is most commonly diagnosed in individuals between the ages of 30 and 40.

5. Other Autoimmune Diseases: Having other autoimmune conditions, such as autoimmune hepatitis or thyroid disease, may increase the risk of PSC.

CLINICAL FEATURES

The clinical presentation of PSC can vary widely, with some patients remaining asymptomatic for years while others develop significant symptoms early in the disease course. Common clinical features of PSC include:

1. Fatigue: Chronic fatigue is a common symptom and can be debilitating for many patients.

2. Pruritus: Severe itching is a frequent complaint and can significantly impact quality of life.

3. Jaundice: Yellowing of the skin and eyes due to elevated bilirubin levels is a hallmark of bile duct obstruction.

4. Abdominal Pain: Pain, typically in the right upper quadrant, may be present due to bile duct inflammation and strictures.

5. Recurrent Cholangitis: Episodes of bacterial infection in the bile ducts can occur, leading to fever, chills, and worsening jaundice.

6. Hepatomegaly and Splenomegaly: Enlargement of the liver and spleen may be noted on physical examination.

7. Portal Hypertension: As the disease progresses, complications related to portal hypertension, such as variceal bleeding and ascites, may develop.

DIAGNOSIS

Diagnosing PSC can be challenging due to its nonspecific symptoms and the need to distinguish it from other liver and bile duct diseases. A combination of clinical evaluation, laboratory tests, imaging studies, and sometimes liver biopsy is used to establish a diagnosis:

1. Medical History and Physical Exam: A thorough medical history and physical examination are essential to identify symptoms, risk factors, and signs of liver disease.

2. Laboratory Tests:

- **Liver Function Tests:** Elevated levels of alkaline phosphatase (ALP) and gamma-glutamyl transferase (GGT) are common in PSC. Bilirubin, AST, and ALT may also be elevated.
- **Autoantibodies:** Tests for autoantibodies, such as antinuclear

antibodies (ANA) and anti-smooth muscle antibodies (ASMA), may be positive but are not specific for PSC.

3. **Imaging Studies:**

- **Magnetic Resonance Cholangiopancreatography (MRCP):** MRCP is the preferred non-invasive imaging modality for diagnosing PSC. It provides detailed images of the bile ducts and can identify characteristic bile duct strictures and dilations.
- **Endoscopic Retrograde Cholangiopancreatography (ERCP):** ERCP can be used for both diagnostic and therapeutic purposes, but it is more invasive than MRCP. It allows direct visualization of the bile ducts and can be used to perform interventions, such as dilation of strictures or stent placement.

4. Liver Biopsy: A liver biopsy may be performed to assess the extent of liver damage and to rule out other liver diseases. The presence of "onion-skin" fibrosis around the bile ducts is a characteristic histological finding in PSC.

MANAGEMENT

At this time, there is no known cure for PSC, and the main approach to treatment is to alleviate symptoms, control the complications and manage the related diseases such as IBD. Management strategies include:

1. Medical Therapy:
- **Ursodeoxycholic Acid (UDCA):** UDCA has been effective in modifying LFT and maybe, has a positive impact on liver but its effects on survival are still unknown.

- **Symptomatic Treatment:** For pruritus, if specific cause cannot be treated, antihistamines or cholestyramine may be given as a medication. Management involving the use of antibiotics is done during episodes of cholangitis.

2. **Endoscopic and Surgical Interventions:**
    - **Endoscopic Therapy:** ERCP can be used to dilate bile duct strictures and place stents to improve bile flow and reduce symptoms.

    - **Surgical Resection:** In some cases, surgical removal of affected bile ducts may be necessary.

    - **Liver Transplantation:** Liver transplantation is the only definitive treatment for end-stage PSC and can be lifesaving. It is considered when liver failure or severe complications occur.

3. Management of Associated Conditions:

- **Inflammatory Bowel Disease (IBD)**: Managing IBD with medications, such as aminosalicylates, immunosuppressants, or biologics, is crucial in patients with PSC and IBD.
- **Colon Cancer Surveillance**: Patients with PSC and IBD are at increased risk for colorectal cancer and should undergo regular colonoscopic surveillance.

7 DAY DIETARY PLAN FOR PSC

Day	Breakfast	Lunch	Dinner
Monday	Oatmeal with berries and a splash of almond milk	Grilled chicken salad with olive oil dressing, whole grain bread	Baked salmon, quinoa, steamed broccoli
Tuesday	Scrambled eggs with spinach and a slice of whole	Lentil soup, mixed green salad and whole grain	Turkey breast, sweet potato, green

	grain toast	crackers	beans
Wednesday	Greek yogurt with honey and a handful of nuts	Quinoa salad with chickpeas, cucumber, tomato, and feta cheese	Grilled chicken breast, brown rice, steamed carrots
Thursday	Smoothie with spinach, banana, and almond milk	Turkey sandwich on whole grain bread, side salad	Baked cod, mashed cauliflower, roasted Brussels sprouts
Friday	Whole grain toast with avocado and a boiled egg	Grilled chicken wrap with veggies and hummus	Baked tofu, wild rice, sautéed spinach
Saturday	Oatmeal with flaxseeds and a splash of almond milk	Baked salmon, barley, steamed asparagus	Lean beef stir-fry with broccoli, carrots, and brown rice
Sunday	Scrambled tofu with veggies	Chicken and vegetable	Grilled shrimp, quinoa,

	and a slice of whole grain toast	stir-fry with brown rice	sautéed green beans

PROGNOSIS

The prognosis of PSC varies widely among individuals and depends on the severity and progression of the disease. Some patients remain asymptomatic or have a slow disease progression, while others may experience rapid deterioration. Factors influencing prognosis include the degree of liver fibrosis, presence of cirrhosis, and development of complications such as cholangiocarcinoma (bile duct cancer), which occurs in about 10-20% of PSC patients.

Despite the lack of a cure, advancements in medical therapy, endoscopic interventions, and liver transplantation have improved the outlook for many PSC patients. Early diagnosis, regular monitoring, and timely intervention are essential to managing the disease and improving quality of life.

CONCLUSION

Liver health is an important factor in people's overall well-being, and proper care for liver disorders entails prompt and accurate diagnosis, appropriate treatment measures, and community awareness. In the case of awareness, prevention, and support of research, the burden experience from liver diseases lessens and, consequently, the quality of life in persons who suffer from these diseases improves. By joining the best efforts and try to mobilize the healthcare providers, investigators, public health organizations, etc, we can get toward the best future which will detect and prevent the liver diseases.

Printed in Great Britain
by Amazon